HEAL WITH NATURAL HERBS®

Enchance your everyday living

D.R. BELL

The contents of this book are presented to help you from beginning to end, from start to finish, and every time you need a friend.

Dear friend, you are not alone.

CreateSpace, an Amazon Company USA

The publication contains the opinions of its author.

The products, information, and use of herbs in this book are not intended to replace, diagnose, treat, prescribe, or contradict the services of a qualified health specialists/physician in the treatment of any aliment/disease. Any application of the information herein is at the reader's discretion and the sole responsibility of the individual who has chosen to use herbal remedies/products. The recipes in this book are intended for adults. Recipes are to be followed exactly as written. The author is not responsible for adverse reactions, or typos. If you have a serious health problem, please consult a competent health practitioner. This information is for educational purposes and should not be used to diagnose or treat diseases.

We do believe that the information is true and correct and was based off many of my travels an research from around the world.

ISBN: 1466384670
ISBN 13: 9781466384675
Library of Congress Control Number: 2011917732
CreateSpace Independent Publishing Platform
North Charleston, South Carolina

Printed in the United States of America.
First Edition

*This book is dedicated to my husband,
Michael A. Bell, my mom, Callie Hawkins,
and my daughter, Ashley R. Hawkins.*

Heal With Natural Herbs®

CONTENTS

Author's Notes · vii

Introduction · ix

Chapter 1 Traditional Chines Medicine (TCM) · · · · · · · 1

Chapter 2 Research Numbers · 4

Chapter 3 Chemically Produced Medications
Have Side Effects · 7

Chapter 4 The Functions of Our Organs · · · · · · · · · · · 11

Chapter 5 Healthy Habits · 13

Chapter 6 Cooking and Cleaning · · · · · · · · · · · · · · · · · 17

Chapter 7 Family Remedies and Recipes · · · · · · · · · · · 18

Chapter 8 Chinese Herbal Medicines in Teas · · · · · · · · 21

Chapter 9 Quotes · 25

Chapter 10 Resources · 28

AUTHOR'S NOTES
BY DENISE R. BELL

DURING MY TRAVELS around the world, my greatest discoveries have been the cultures of other people, their different ways of life, and the many amazing alternative methods of healing available on our earth. Thankfully, a different interest has developed in me, one for Chinese herbal medication, which has been practiced for centuries.

Through using Traditional Chines Medicine (TCM), eating healthy food, and exercising regularly, I have actually healed myself and according to my medical records, my health has improved. You, too, can live a healthier, happier life for good. You can free yourself from pollutions and take the simple steps towards the goals of an alternative, healthy life.

Stay determined, devoted, disciplined, and full of desire so that this renowned healthy way of life can help you maintain a balanced life. Heal to be healthy.

Heal with Natural Herbs® is my gift of knowledge to you.

INTRODUCTION

ARE YOU TIRED of being misdiagnosed? Are you on a diet and bogged down with charts, quick-acting weight loss pills, and calorie counting but still don't have a clue what it takes to obtain and maintain good health? Are you currently taking expensive medications that have side effects? If you answered yes to one or more of these questions, this book is for you. Using natural herbs will enhance your everyday life. If you use the proper herbs and teas, and engage in positive diet and exercise, you will be initiated into a healthy transformation that your body very much deserves. **Remember, no impurities grow in pure blood.** Those awful side effects from prescription drugs can cause uric acid buildup in the body. Mucus and acid are harmful to the body. Infection is made up of parasites that invade a body part of tissue and can lead to disease. The three-thousand-year-old practice of Traditional Chinese Medicine, TCM, has been known to have medicinal healing properties, but remember to always use TCM safely and effectively. **Start Purifying now!**

Throughout its chapters, Healing with Natural Herbs will discuss how to be aware of your body's functions, and how TCM works with your body. You will learn to use natural herbs to help control disease. Quotes, recipes, and tips for developing healthy living habits abound in this book. If you are already healthy and want an alternative solution to staying healthy, this book will explain good healing properties. You will also learn how to rid your body of toxic waste using old-fashioned healing recipes, and find out how to purchase the TCM products that made my body complete and rejuvenated. I hope that this book will be a guide for you in maintaining a healthier, happier, normal life. Enhance your life.

CHAPTER 1

TRADITIONAL CHINES MEDICINE (TCM)

"For every ailment that we know, nature
allows for an herb to grow."
—UNKNOWN

CHINESE KNOWLEDGE, TRADITIONS, and dynasties have been evolving since 2100 BC. One of the greatest of the Chinese medicine men, Hu Tuo, lived from 141-208 AD and was known to treat tumors on the skin. Sun Simaio (581-682 AD) said that good habits, such as eating a wholesome diet, exercising, and having sex on a regular basis would give you longevity. Simaio died at the age of one hundred and one. Zhang Zhong Jin (150-219 ad) created a chart to indicated the positions used in acupuncture. Acupuncture is an alternative medicine that threats the patient thought the insertion of needles into the body. Li Shizhen (1517-1593 AD) listed two thousand herbal medicines. His interest was in science and Western medical studies.

Traditional Chinese Medicine has been used for a long period of time, dating back centuries. Certain plants were first used for cooking purposes in making soups, stews, teats, and several other culinary dishes. It was then discovered that some of the planted being used has different effects on the body, such as healing, drowsiness, diarrhea, and other sicknesses. Later, it was determined that some plants had the medicinal potential to actually heal though reducing skin tumors, relieving the pain caused by headaches and various other pains of the body, and treating other related ailments. Some of the herbs helped patients to have a quicker recovery from sickness. Wood Betony helps the nervous system. Rhubarb helps stimulates the liver and helps relieve constipation. **Avoid Rhubarb when pregnant**, though as it is a very strong purgative. **Attention:** Herbs have a tendency to expel toxins from the body's system that may have been causing your disease. Healing stemming from Traditional Chinese Medicine tends to be permanent. We will discuss herbs and their properties in Chapter Eight. Be aware of your body's functions and how they work. Chinese herbs will help you maintain a happier, healthier life, such as with the use of a high-potency full-body cleansing teat that is available for purchase thought our website at www.healingwithnaturalherbs.com. Take the initiative to make a new, health-conscious decision.

NATURAL HERBS: HOW CAN YOU LIVE WITHOUT THEM?
Homeopathy is the use of a specific type of preparation consisting of several substances, and it is considered a natural remedy. Traditional Chinese Medicine doesn't use substances besides plants, and is intended to help the immune system to fight on its own. TCM also doesn't use diluted substances like homeopathy does. Remember, herbs are natural so they will take time to work. Most of us want instant gratification but natural herbs will not work overnight. If you have the patience, you will surely see worthwhile results. Using and maintaining alterative healing with natural herbs works wonders. **It is not against the law to doctor yourself.**

Traditional Chinese Medicine is a renowned way of life that will help you maintain a balanced life. Therefore, if you have the desire, devotion, dedication, and discipline, you will experience positive results. Dear friend, you're not alone. **<u>Quit ignoring your body's systems and improve your life-you deserve it.</u>**

CHAPTER 2

RESEARCH NUMBERS

"The fruit of the tree was for the man's meat
and the [leaves] for the man's healing."
—EZEKIEL 47:12

ACCORDING TO DATA gathered by the American Institute for Cancer Research (AICR), there will be about 201,090 new cases of invasive breast cancer diagnosed in women, by 2030 the top cancer that will be diagnosed will be breast, prostate and lung the study finds, and about 785,000 Americans will have their first heart attack. Also, while 203,415 men develop prostate cancer, 28,370 men will die from it. Over 100,000 cancers are linked to excessive body fat. Are you aware that nearly 24 million people in the United States have diabetes? And according to the American Stroke Society, about 795,000 Americans each year suffer from a stroke. A stroke happens every forty seconds. On average, every four minutes a person dies from a stroke.

There are also a variety of different infections that are commonly misdiagnosed. Infection can lead to disease.

Some infections may be easily overlooked, such as an ear infection, which can then lead to fever, diarrhea, chills, and nausea. Another potentially overlooked infection is an abscessed took, whose symptoms include pus that settled in the jaw.

Don't' forget that honesty and being true to yourself is the most important part of making your life happier and more loving. Consider that you have a chance, and you will soon have the knowledge to utilize the leaves that were put on this earth to medicinally health and help all mankind. **Attention: Life begins in the colon and death ends in the colon!** Toxic buildup may cause cancer in the intestines after years of toxemia and constipation. Some symptoms of toxic buildup that you may not be aware of include:

- Sinus colds and flu
- Prostate troubles
- Lack of sexual desire
- Gas, belching, or flatus
- Depression, fatigue
- Cough, shortness of breath

Other symptoms of sickness may be related to stress, obesity, overeating, and the immune system being compromised.

Just think of all the bad sugars that are still in your body from all the years of unhealthy eating you've done. During a person's lifetime, the digestive system processes 60,000 to 100,000 pounds of food. Just imagine how much of that food is still in your colon if you're not eliminating it regularly. An adult's intestines are usually twenty-seven feet long and it usually takes a meal fifteen hours to two days to completely pass through it. The pancreas helps control and balance the digestive system.

Keep in mind cancer can't grow in a healthy organ; so getting rid of toxins is a healthy decision.

CHAPTER 3

CHEMICALLY PRODUCED MEDICATIONS HAVE SIDE EFFECTS

"To administer medicines for illness which have already developed is akin to the conduct of a man who begins to dig a well after he has become thirsty."
—THE INTERNAL BOOK OF HUANG DI

NO INSURANCE, MISDIAGNOSED, losing existing coverage. Are you scared you are going to hear these terrifying words? Will the treatment do more harm than good? You might be thinking, do I really need additional tests, and am I really hearing the truth from a trustworthy physician or nurse practitioner? Why do I trust someone to give me chemically produced medicines that have a lot of side effects? For the most part, these chemically produced medicines can do more harm than good. At one time or another, did you or someone you confided in to make a health decision for you make you feel fearful? Maybe at some point they even pressured you and your loved ones to make quick decisions that may or may not have had positive results. Maybe at that time you were not aware of a second option, of an alternative way of living that may be better for you: Traditional Chinese Medicine.

Compare your everyday side effects and the prices of chemically produced drugs to natural herbs. Natural herbs lead to a better way of life than chemicals. The average cost of prescription drugs for twenty to thirty milligrams, filled in quantities of ninety to one hundred capsules (the count may vary), can be very pricey, potentially costing you hundreds of dollars for one prescription bottle of pills. These chemically produced drugs can cause serious side effects and may even cause death. Please thread the insert before you consume any pills that may harm you.

"Pills are bills."
—CALLIE HAWKINS

For over three thousand years, the Chinese have been using natural herbal medicine, and they have accumulated an impressive breath of knowledge of remedies and medicinal healing. Learn the facts so you will not be at a disadvantage when it comes to decisions about your health. If you continue to put chemicals in your body, you will be prone to disease. The fruits were made to be eaten; the leaves were put on this earth for medicinal purposes.

"Our greatest glory is not in never falling but in getting back up every time we do."
—CONFUCIUS

Some of your symptoms may have gone unnoticed, or you may not be able to recognize them. No need to be scared! Detect and correct. Who wants to be sick? The use of Traditional Chinese Medicine can help control symptoms such as diarrhea, stomach ulcers, intestinal parasites, bad breath, bloating, and gas. It can also help with the following internal disorders: diabetes, cancer, high cholesterol, headaches, immune system functions, and kidney and bladder problems. Women's issues such as intense menstrual cramps, irregular menstrual flow, and other related conditions may also be helped with Traditional Chinese medicine. A lack of sexual desire in men, impotency, and premature ejaculation may also be helped. Using natural herbs could also help with addictions to drugs, alcohol, and sugar. Upper respiratory system conditions such as colds, coughs, sinus infections, asthma, and throat infections may be caused by sore throat, toothache, and gingivitis and may be helped by TCM. Some skin infections such as psoriasis, eczema, and boils-as well as muscular issues such as arthritis, back pain, fibromyalgia, and sore muscles-can all be helped using Traditional Chinese Medicine.

Now that you understand some of the symptoms that you may have ignored or never noticed before, you are ready to correct them. Herbal medicine has been around for a long period of time. It is not against the law to be able to recognized unusual symptoms. Have you really and truly read the inserts that come with the medications that you are prescribed? The last insert that I read included the following possible side effects: bleeding, mental changes, red skin or blistering, trouble breathing, and swollen and/or pealing skin. **It is not against the law to use your own personal judgment**, although you should use it wisely. Obtain as much information as you can so you aren't misled.

According to data from the American College of Radiology, in 2004, noted on the website insurance-fraud. org, some doctors request additional tests that may be unnecessary. Numerous requests for tests have possibly reduced malpractice suits. It was also reported that some doctors have been known to bill insurance companies to see how much they can overcharge while still receiving payment. Overcharging for services that have not been rendered can lead to claims of fraud. Medicare and private health insurers pay up to $16 billion a year for needless imaging tests that have been ordered by doctors.

Don't continue to suffer from a lack of knowledge. My friend, we are here and will be supportive of each other. Taking care of your body should be part of your daily ritual. Now is a good time to take your health care to a more aggressive level. Expel those toxins with High Potency Five Day Cleansing Tea. Confucius once said, "In life, bad news is always followed by good news." The bad news is that we have been eating unhealthy foods most of our lives. The good news is that we can start being healthy now. In a later chapter we will discuss better eating habits, exercise, and TCM's healing properties and teas.

CHAPTER 4

THE FUNCTIONS OF OUR ORGANS

"The greatest cure for any disease is nutritional foods that feed the specific need."
—ROY HOWARD

FIRST THING'S FIRST, let's get a better understanding of our body and how to listen for unusual symptoms, so that you will be aware of anything that could be detrimental to your health. The human body has ten main organs: brain, lungs, heart, stomach, intestines, liver, pancreas, kidneys, bowels, and skin.

- The brain is the center of the nervous system and is surrounded by the cranium. It is attached to the spinal cord and relies on various joints. The brain controls thoughts, memory, and speech.
- The lungs are essential to the respiratory system. Humans have two lungs, the left being divided into two lobes and the right into three. The lungs carry oxygen to the bloodstream.
- The heart is a myogenic organ that carries oxygen to the organs. The heart works like a pump.

- The stomach is a muscular, hollow, dilated part of the alimentary canal that can store up to two-and-a-half pints of food. Your stomach is located under your diaphragm on the left side of the abdomen.
- The intestines move food particles from the small to the large intestines. Some digestion takes place in the intestines; however, the remaining waste exits though the anus.
- The liver produces bile, which breaks down fat in the intestines.
- The pancreas carries digestive fluids to the duodenum, or the first part of the small intestine.
- The kidneys are very close to the spine, with the adrenal glands on top of them. They are responsible for filtering your blood.
- The bowel is the canal extending from the pyloric sphincter of the stomach to the anus.
- The skin is the largest organ of your body, and it is made up of two layers; the epidermis is on the surface and the dermis is underneath.

Take a deep breath. Don't you feel better already? Now that you know what the basic organ functions are, how could you not want a true healthy life with TCM? Chinese herbs help maintain a healthy body and a happier you. Are you ready to begin healing?

> *"Everybody wants to be healthy, but*
> *no one wants to give it a try."*
> —DENISE R. BELL

CHAPTER 5

HEALTHY HABITS

*"It's not the food in your life, but the life
in your food that nourishes you."*
—MARK AT CHARLES GORDON MARKET,
MONTEGO BAY, JAMAICA

FRUITS AND VEGETABLES should be a part of your everyday life. Try to eat what's in season. Make healthy snacks ahead of time and store them either in the refrigerator or in a cool place. Healthy snacks can be raw vegetables, fresh fruits, dry cereal, or whatever you like. Fresh strawberries are a good example of a snack that can be put into a sandwich bag. Snacks made ahead of time will help you have more productive and less stressful week. Eat a healthy snack in the morning as you are headed for work or school; let this be your daily ritual. Your body is in much need of nutritional healing. Keep your body energized. Plus, just imagine all the money you'll save. A penny saved is a penny earned.

When you add more fruits and vegetables to your diet, you are getting healthy doses of Vitamin C and other vitamins. And guess what? Fruits and vegetables are low in calories. You are truly on your way to understanding how crucial a healthy lifestyle is.

Ask yourself, do I need a lot of confusing charges and quick weigh loss diet plans to stay healthy? The fact is that I have never known a chart that has made me healthy. The insanity of it all is that you keep destroying your body and expecting it to heal by itself. Now that you have come to terms with the need to have a healthy body, you can change your diet to a healthier way of eating and realize that there is no need to endlessly counting calories anymore. For the most part, vegetables have very low calories in them. It's the life in your food that nourishes you.

Eat live foods or raw foods, such as carrots, green peppers, and leafy green vegetables. You can eat them fresh out of the garden without changing the texture by blending and missing them. Eating live foods will help to expel that pasty fecal matter that may be obstructing your colon and causing acute or chronic diseases. High Potency Five Day Cleaning Tea can also help promote a healthy bladder, liver, and colon, all in one.

Eat live foods that are uncooked and unprocessed, so that you will get the enzymes that your body needs. Cooking foods at temperatures higher than 104 degrees Fahrenheit often destroys the enzymes that help break down food during digestion.

People are watching more of what they eat in today's society. The Raw Movement is seeing more people buying and eating locally grown foods. Chinese cabbage is a natural herb also referred to as bok choy and has excellent healing properties that can reduce cataracts and some cancers. Oranges help relieve coughs, remove phlegm from the throat, and calm the nerves. Trader Joe's, HEB, Sprouts, Kroger, and Whole Foods are good markets in which to buy organic produce and gluten-free meals.

Growing your own food is a good way to make sure that you are getting the best nutritional value. It is a healthy alternative to eating genetically altered foods that can harm the liver, raise your cholesterol, and may cause cancer.

"We eat what we grow."
—MARK, MONTEGO BAY JAMAICA

When you eat nourishing food, your body tends to have more energy, and your attention span is a lot longer. In most cases your completion is a lot clearer as well. When you eat unhealthy, you look unhealthy. Because of the poor eating habits that we have developed over the years, ou8r bodies are reacting to a feast-or-famine scenario: I don't know when you are going to feed me again, so I am going to store some fat for later. Often what makes us change our eating habits is an unexpected health issue-such as a stroke or heart attack-that could have ended in death.

Exercise will also help keep the doctor away and reduce illness. Regular exercise is important. Try Tai Chi, which is a soft style of martial arts using slow movements.

Yoga and meditation go hand-in-hand. It relieves stress, improves your health, and strengthens your body. Yoga also relaxes and calms, keeping you focused and in a better state of mind. Swimming is one of the ultimate exercises a person can try. You work every body part without a high impact workout. Healthy eating habits can change your libido. With Traditional Chinese Medicine, healing starts by releasing the chemical poisons from your bloodstream that can cause your body to be septic. Promise yourself that you will practice healthy living in your everyday life. More than likely you will feel more confident and feel much better overall, and you will look better too! Taking care of your body should be a daily ritual. Now it's a good time to take your health care to a more aggressive level, especially in today's society.

CHAPTER 6

COOKING AND CLEANING

*"Our greatest glory is not in never failing but
in getting back up every time we do."*
—CONFUCIUS

USE STAINLESS STEEL cooking pots and pans. No poisonous gasses can be released from stainless steel pans to enter into your bloodstream. Back cast iron skillets can also be used. Cast iron skillets cook evenly, holding the desire heath, and have a lower change of E. coli contamination. **Warning:** Use oven gloves that can resist up to 400 Fahrenheit when handling cast iron, as it tends to get very hot.

Clean your uncooked meat in lemon juice and let it marinate until thawed. The citric acid in the lemon juice cleans the meat better than running it under tap water. Wash your dishes in warm to hot water with a dash of bleach. Bleach kills germs. Pour a dash of bleach in your bath water when you come home from sleeping in different beds that may have bed bugs. Bleach kills the bugs.

CHAPTER 7

FAMILY REMEDIES AND RECIPES

THE FOLLOWING RECIPES are some of my family's recipes that my mother remembers from childhood. For the most part, these remedies have been used by African descendants from the Caribbean. My mother is seventy-six years old, uses Traditional Chinese Medicine, and has no known life-threatening diseases.

Visualize a grandmotherly woman in the kitchen cooking up some kind of tonic, infusion, or decoction to help make somebody feel better. She has multiple stainless steel pots bubbling on the stove, as steam and strong vapors fill the air with medicinal scents. Back in the day, some people had extensive knowledge about home remedies, and they were very educated in herbal principals and how to use herbs in tonics, tinctures, and ointments. Centuries ago, people relied on almanacs, the constellations, sundials, and other down-to-earth tools in their daily lives. More recently, my mother remember the days when doctors would make house calls and people used home remedies to heal, cook, and clean.

- **Aunt Carol's Calmer**
  One teaspoon of lime juice will help calm those hyper chaps (kids). It also helps with colds and breaks down fat. Aunt Carol noticed that her great nieces got better sleep after taking lime.
- **MB Trapped Gas**
  Lay on your back, thrust your knees to the middle of your chest, and the pressure will be released.
- **Remove Toxic Smells**
  Strike a match. Once it is lit, blow out the match and those toxic smells will disappear.
- **Sea Salt Bath**
  Pour one cup of sea salt into bath water. Make sure the temperature is nice and warm. Seas salt cleans the skin, which is the largest organ of your body.
- **Aldine's Tummy Toxin Lifter**
  Hold one or two tablespoons of coconut oil in your mouth for at least five minutes without swallowing. Spit it out and discard of it properly. You may repeat the process every five minutes for fifteen minutes. The coconut oil cleanses toxins from your stomach through the help of the saliva glands.
- **Ollie's Lavender Mouthwash**
  Mix half a bottle of distilled water with half a teaspoon of lavender. Shake very well and gargle. Do not swallow.
- **Goldie's Gargle (sore throat)**
  Mix one fresh squeezed lemon with half a teaspoon of salt and two ounces of apple cider vinegar. Mix

thoroughly and gargle. Do not swallow. This mixture should help remove mucous.

- **Mother Nature's Fever Reducer**
  Use a big container and fill with cold, distilled water. Add once ounce of white vinegar. Immerse the washcloths in the solution, and let them soak for a minute. Wring out washcloths and place them on the neck, breast, head, armpits, and inner thighs of the person with high fever. Make sure the person is not smothered in hot covers. Leave cold packs on. As the person warms up, turn him or her, and you will notice that the fever has transferred to the washcloths. Add ice or change water. Repeat until the fever has gone down, and then put dry clothes on your patient.

- **Organic Pure Honey**
  Add honey to your teas and other drinks. Honey is a source of energy.

- **Hot Flashes**
  Sip (one Tsp.) Apple Cider Vinegar use as needed, but don't over do it.

CHINESE HERBAL MEDICINES IN TEAS

HIGH POTENCY FIVE Day Cleansing Tea consists of 100 percent natural products, with no chemical fillers. The natural herbs in the tea help promote healthy blood vessels and eliminate toxins in the liver, intestines, and bladder. Teas also help with dissolving kidney stones, the retention of urine, and cleaning the bladder. Here is a list of some supportive natural herbs that are found in teas.

Hawthorn: It is used as an herbal remedy to treat constipation and heart and liver problems. Hawthorn is part of the rose family and has the medicinal value of being rich in flavonoids and antioxidants.

Tree of Heaven: This tree grows very rapidly in China and has reached heights of eighty feet. It has a smooth gray bark, and it is considered a natural antibiotic. Its medicinal purposes include helping to prevent skin cancer and promoting health in the heart, blood vessels, and skin. It has been used for epilepsy, heart issues, tapeworms, and malaria.

Green Tangerine: This helps promote a healthy liver, bladder, and colon.

Thorough Wax: This is also known as licorice root and Korean ginseng. This herb is good for hepatitis, reducing the symptoms of PMS, lowering inflammation, and curing skin infections; it also helps strengthen the muscles. In TCM, it is known to help with congestion and respiratory problems.

Skull Cap: This is a plant that has been around for centuries. It promotes healthy nerves and is good for anxiety and hormone imbalance.

Plantago Seed: Plantago helps with bladder problems, unhealthy blood sugar, high cholesterol, kidney function, hypertension, skin inflammation, and malignant ulcers. It is safe and effective for bleeding.

These six natural herbs are used in the High Potency Five Day Cleansing Tea to help promote healthy kidneys, liver, and colon, as well as the above mentioned remedies. Herbal teas help control allergies, arthritis, gout, high blood pressure, impotency, headaches, migraines, diabetes, thyroid, tumors, fibroid tumors, hormone imbalance, cholesterol, hepatitis (A, B, and C), and the cells that may cause cancer.

Treat minor ailments immediately so they won't have a chance to develop into acute, chronic, or even incurable conditions.

What is a herb? A herb is any flower or plant with a stem and root. It can also be used in medicine or cooking. Herbs have been dyed back over 3000 B.C.

Some herbs can be used for medicinal healing.

Aloe Vera: Purifier also rich in calcium, potassium and Vitamin B-12. It cleanses the kidneys, bladder and removes fecal matter from the colon. Aloe stimulates hair growth, and kills bacterial that may cause scalp disease.

Avocado: Avocados are rich in protein, Vitamin A, B, C D, E and Chlorophyll and Iron. Avocados help your digestive system. The Avocado seed contains an antibiotic that will kill rats when mixed with cheese.

Cannabis: (Sativa) popular names are also called marijuana, pot, and ganja. Cannabis has medicinal healing. Cannabis can be made as a poultice to help ulcers, boils, and infections to help kill pain.

Chamomile: (manzilla) known herb for relaxing the nerves and relieving muscle pain.

Dandelion: flowers rich in Vitamin C and D. Dandelion helps obstruct the spleen, liver, and bladder, and remove excess mucus.

Flax: Also known as linseed. Flax is rich in calcium, potassium, magnesium. Flax has medicinal purposes. A decoction can help relieve menstrual cramps, coughs, urinary tract disorders, and lung. '

Garlic: It is a purifier and helps control high blood pressure. Garlic has been known to help a cough.

Ginger: Stimulates your appetite. It helps detox waste from the skin. It can be used in teas.

Honey: Natural sweetener. Honey is good in teas. Honey has medicinal purposes such as constipation.

Mango: It is a source of Vitamin A and other vitamins. Mangos can help hypertension and fever.

Peppermint: It is used in teas to help the stomach. It can also be used to calm nerves and lower blood pressure.

CHAPTER 9

QUOTES

SOME OF THE quotes that you have read throughout the book are helpful in remaining focused on the healing process.

"Pills make bills."
—CALLIE HAWKINS

"The fruit of the tree was for man's meat and the [leaves] for man's healing."
—EZEKIEL 47:12

"Our greatest glory is not in never falling but in getting up every time we do."
—CONFUCIUS

"The greatest cure for any disease is nutritional foods that feed the specific need."
—ROY HOWARD

*"For every ailment that we know, nature
allows for an herb to grow."*
—UNKNOWN

"We eat what we grow."
—MARK, MONTEGO BAY, JAMAICA

"In life, band news is always followed by good news."
—CONFUCIUS

*"It's not the food in your life, but the life
in your food that nourishes you."*
—MARK AT CHARLES GORDON MARKET, MONTEGO BAY, JAMAICA

*"To administer medicines for illness which have
already developed is akin to the conduct of a man who
begins to dig a well after he has become thirsty."*
—THE INTERNAL BOOK OF HUANG DI

*"Treat hot illnesses with cool medicines and
cold illnesses with warm medicines."*
—THE PHARMACOPEIA OF SHEN NONG

*"Heal to be healthy. Everybody wants to be
healthy, but no one wants to give it a try."*
—D.R. BELL

These are a few quotes that have kept my journey positive and motivating. My history of using herbs to heal dates back to when I was a teenager.

Need a healing?

Mother Nature has always been here. Where have you been?

Natural herbs: How can you live without them?

Take time to stay healthy!

This book is available with quantity discounts for bulk purchases when used to promote product information. Visit our website at www.healwithnaturalherbs.com to see our teas and other future products that will be available so that you may live healthy. Our official trademark medicinal T-shirt is also available for **ORDER NOW! @healwithnaturalherbs.com**

Follow us on Twitter, Fb, You Tube, Instagram, Tumblr

Buy our products on Amazonhealwithnaturalherbs

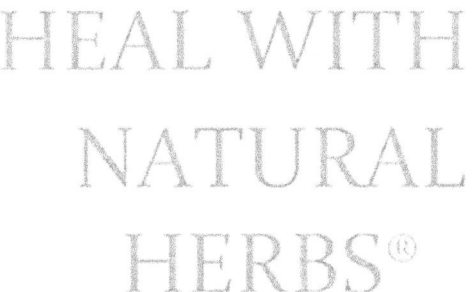

HEAL WITH NATURAL HERBS®

CHAPTER 10

RESOURCES

Hawthorne Frail
En. Wikidedia.org
Institute of Traditional Medicine Opine
Keo, Erl-Shyh; Wong, C.j.; Lin, W.L.; Chu, C.V.; Tsen, T.N.;
Chau-Jong Wang; Wes-Lung Lin, Lin, chia- Yih Chu, Tsui-
Hua Tseng (2007)

Effects of polyphenois derived from fruit of crotaegus
pinnatfda on cell transformation dermal edema and skin
tumor formations by phorbol ester application.

American Cancer Society
http://www.cancer.org

American Heart Society
Heart and Stroke Information (800) AHA-USA1
http://www.americanheart.org

The Herb Research Foundation
http://herbs.org

National Center for Homeopathy
http://healthy.net/neh/nch/index.html

Medical Dictionary: Medline Plus-National Library of Medicine
http://www.nlm.nih.gov/medlineplus/mplusdictionary.org

Order Now!

Live An Improved Life. You Deserve It.

Or Write to us at:
Mothernature Natural Herbs
P.O. Box 3815
Humble, Texas 77347-3815
info@healwithnaturalherbs.com
www.healwithnaturalherbs.com

"Healing with Natural herbs should be a way of life.
Heal to Healthy."